Keto Bread Every Day

Healthy and Low Carb Recipes Perfect for Any Occasion

Sarah James

TABLE OF CONTENTS

INTRODUCTION

Keto bread is a low-carbohydrate, high-fat liquid diet plan that requires you to consume a lot of healthy fats through either a keto bread recipe book or diet program. It's short for the controversial low-carbohydrate ketogenic diet more commonly referred to as the ketogenic diet. There are many variations of the keto diet with different levels of restrictions. For example, some people may only get 20 grams of carbohydrates per day while others restrict their intake to 5 grams of carbohydrates per day. The keto diet can be used as a short term diet, but most people choose to follow it for more than a month.

How Does Keto Bread Help You Lose Weight?

The idea behind the keto bread diet is that when you eat lots of healthy fats such as butter, olive oil, avocados, macadamia nuts, eggs, and grass-fed meats you will lose weight quickly and easily. The key to losing weight fast with this kind of eating plan is to take in so many calories through fat that you end up burning off the extra calories you burned from food intake. The keto bread diet plan isn't hard to follow if you stick to the rules. It's just a matter of cutting out most carbs and eating lots of healthy fats.

Is Eating Keto Bread Right For You?

If you want to lose weight fast and lose it completely with no chance of gaining it back then the keto bread recipe book or ketogenic diet might be right for you. It's not right for everyone though and can't be used in place of other methods like exercise and eating less food on your own as part of your weight loss program. If you're going to use this kind of eating plan make sure you check w/ your doctor first to see if it's right for you before putting it into action

The Keto diet has become more popular in the last few years. It is a low-carb, high-fat eating style that has been highly researched and proven to be effective. Here at Keto Bread, we have all of the necessary tools for anyone who is interested in changing their eating patterns to something healthier, such as the Men's Standard Keto Cookbook. We understand that everyone's nutritional needs are different, so we have cataloged a wide variety of recipes to meet your needs. Keto is a deficient carbohydrate diet with ample protein, which is allowed during the diet. It is not just a ketogenic change in the diet and grows healthy eating habits.

They create healthy and natural eating habits for you stronger both physically and mentally. Our body needs energy as it is coming from carbohydrates; our body uses glucose (carbohydrates) as a primary energy source.

The ketogenic diet is a low-calorie, high-fat diet in which fat is converted into energy instead of glucose. During this process, fatty acids are released from your body, and our liver renovates these fatty acids into ketones. When ketone levels have increased in the blood goes to the brain and replaces glucose with energy. You can reach this stage in the first week of the ketogenic diet.

The keto diet is not new, but its popularity has declined over time as various medical developments seem to help with conditions like epilepsy and weight loss. However, now, people are again beginning to see it as a way to lose weight, lighten skin, maintain their health, and even live longer. So much to wait for!

Our body uses glucose as its primary source of energy. Never Carbohydrates are metabolized, and glucose is produced in our body. This glucose is stored in the cells of our body. When glucose levels rise, then the excess glucose is converted to glycogen. This chemical process of the conversion of glucose to glycogen is called glycogenesis. This glycogen is stored in the muscles of the body and liver as a backup source of energy. In this diet, your body undergoes many adjustments. Some different signs and symptoms confirm that you are in ketosis.

BASIC BREAD

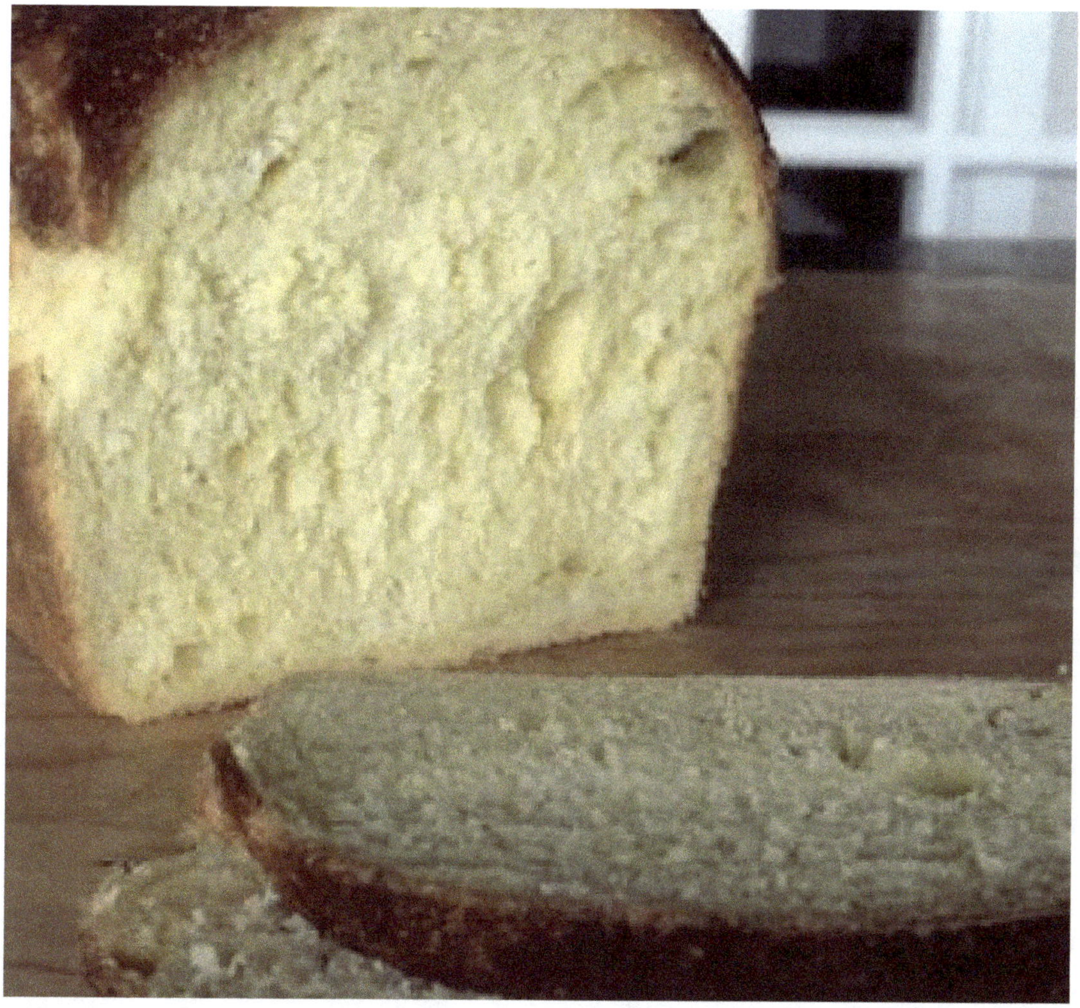

CHEESE SAUSAGE BREAD

Preparation time: 4 hours

Cooking time: 4 hours

Servings: 8

Ingredients:

1 teaspoon dry yeast

3 ½ cups flour

1 teaspoon salt

1 tablespoon sugar

1 cup water

1 ½ tablespoon oil

2 tablespoons smoked sausage

2 tablespoons grated cheese

1 tablespoon chopped garlic

Directions:

Cut the sausage into small cubes. Grate the cheese on a grater; chop the garlic.

Add the ingredients to the bread machine according to the instructions.

Turn on the baking program, and let it do the work.

Nutrition:

Carbohydrates: 4 g | Fats: 5.6 g | Proteins: 7.7 g | Calories: 260 | Fibers: 1.3 g

LEMON BLUEBERRY BREAD

Preparation time: 2 hours

Cooking time: 25 minutes

Servings: 10

Ingredients:

2 cups almond flour

1/2 cup coconut flour

1/2 cup ghee

1/2 cup coconut oil, melted

1/2 cup erythritol | 4 eggs

2 tablespoons lemon zest, about half a lemon

1 teaspoon lemon juice

1/2 cup blueberries

2 teaspoons baking powder

Directions:

Lightly beat eggs before pouring them into your bread machine pan.

Add in melted coconut oil, ghee, and lemon juice to the pan.

Add the remaining dry ingredients including blueberries and lemon zest to the bread machine pan. Set bread machine to quick bread setting.

When the bread is done, remove the bread machine pan from the bread machine.

Let it cool slightly before transferring to a cooling rack.

You can store your bread for up to 5 days.

Nutrition:

Calories: 300| Carbohydrates: 14 g | Proteins: 5 g | Fats: 30 g

SWEET COFFEE BREAD

Preparation time: 2 hours

Cooking time: 25 minutes

Servings: 10

Ingredients:

2 cups of almond fine flour

½ teaspoon salt | 4 eggs

Cinnamon, three-quarters of a teaspoon

½ cup swerve Keto sweetener

½ cup of unsalted melted butter

¼ cup of protein powder that is not flavored

4 teaspoons of coconut flour

2/3 cup of almond milk that is not sweetened

2 teaspoons espresso

½ teaspoon extract from vanilla

2 teaspoons active dry yeast

2 teaspoons baking powder

Directions:

Mix together the almond flour, coconut flour, sweetener swerve, cinnamon, salt, baking powder, espresso, and unflavored protein powder in a container.

Mix the unsweetened almond milk, eggs, extract of vanilla, and unsalted melted butter in another container. As per the instructions on the manual of your machine, pour the ingredients in the bread pan, taking care to follow how to mix in the yeast.

Place the bread pan in the machine, and select the sweet bread setting, together with the crust type, if available, then press Start once you have closed the lid of the machine.

When the bread is ready, extract it from the pan and place it on a wire mesh surface to cool before cutting it.

Nutrition: Calories: 177.7 | Fats: 3.8 g | Carbs: 31 g | Proteins: 4.6 g

BREAD WITH BEEF

Preparation time: 2 hours

Cooking time: 2 hours

Servings: 6

Ingredients:

5 oz. beef | 15 oz. almond flour

5 oz. rye flour | 1 onion

3 teaspoons dry yeast

5 tablespoons olive oil

1 tablespoon sugar

Sea salt | Ground black pepper

Directions:

Pour the warm water into the 15 oz. of the wheat flour and rye flour and leave overnight.

Chop the onions and cut the beef into cubes. Fry the onions until clear and golden brown and then mix in the bacon and fry on low heat for 20 minutes until soft.

Combine the yeast with the warm water, mixing until smooth consistency, and then combine the yeast with the flour, salt and sugar, but don't forget to mix and knead well.

Add in the fried onions with the beef and black pepper and mix well. Pour some oil into a bread machine and place the dough into the bread maker.

Cover the dough with the towel and leave for 1 hour. Close the lid and turn the bread machine on the basic/white bread program.

Bake the bread until the medium crust and after the bread is ready take it out and leave for 1 hour covered with the towel and only then you can slice the bread.

Nutrition:

Carbohydrates: 6 g | Fats: 21 g | Proteins: 13 g | Calories: 299 | Fibers: 1.6 g

CINNAMON CAKE

Preparation time: 7 minutes

Cooking time: 5 minutes

Servings: 12

Ingredients:

½ cup erythritol | ½ cup butter

½ tablespoon vanilla extract

1 ¾ cups almond flour

1 ½ teaspoon baking powder

1 ½ teaspoon cinnamon

¼ teaspoon sea salt

1 ½ cup carrots, grated

1 cup pecans, chopped

Directions:

Grate carrots and place them in a food processor. Add in the rest of the ingredients, except the pecans, and process until well incorporated. Fold in pecans.

Pour mixture into bread machine pan. Set bread machine to bake.

When baking is completed, remove from the bread machine and transfer to a cooling rack.

Allow cooling completely before slicing. (You can also top with a sugar-free cream cheese frosting, see recipe below).

You can store for up to 5 days in the refrigerator.

Nutrition:

Calories: 350 | Carbohydrates: 8 g | Fats: 34 g | Proteins: 7 g

GREAT FLAVOR CHEESE BREAD WITH THE ADDED KICK OF PIMENTO OLIVES

Preparation time: 5 minutes

Cooking time: 3 hours

Servings: 1 loaf

Ingredients:

1 cup water room temperature

4 teaspoons sugar

3/4 teaspoon salt

1 ¼ cups shredded sharp Cheddar cheese

3 cups bread flour

2 teaspoons active dry yeast

3/4 cup pimiento olives, drained and sliced

Directions:

Add all ingredients except olives to the machine pan.

Select basic bread setting.

At prompt before second knead, mix in olives.

Nutrition:

Calories: 124 | Total Fats: 4 g | Carbs: 19 g | Fibers: 1 g | Proteins: 5 g

WILD RICE CRANBERRY BREAD

Preparation time: 5 minutes

Cooking time: 3 hours

Servings: 1 loaf

Ingredients:

1 ¼ cup water

¼ cup skim milk powder

1 ¼ teaspoon salt

2 tablespoons liquid honey

1 tablespoon extra-virgin olive oil

3 cups all-purpose flour

3/4 cup cooked wild rice

1/4 cup pine nuts

¾ teaspoon celery seeds

1/8 teaspoon freshly ground black pepper

1 teaspoon bread machine or instant yeast

2/3 cup dried cranberries

Directions:

Add all ingredients to the machine pan except the cranberries.

Place pan into the oven chamber. Select Basic bread setting.

At the signal to add ingredients, add the cranberries.

Nutrition:

Calories: 225 | Total Fats: 7.8 g | Carbs: 33 g | Fibers: 1 g | Proteins: 6.7 g

FANTASTIC BREAD

Preparation time: 5 minutes

Cooking time: 20 minutes

Servings: 6

Ingredients:

1 cup almond flour or almond supper

4 tablespoons entire psyllium husk

2 teaspoons of preparing powder

1/2 teaspoon of salt (discretionary)

little bunch almond fragments (discretionary)

little bunch squashed pecans

6 large eggs | 1 cup full-fat yogurt

Directions:

Add the dry ingredients to a big blending bowl and mix. The nuts are discretionary or can fill in for different kinds of nuts on the off chance that you like.

Crack 6 large eggs into a different blending bowl, add one cup full-fat yogurt, and blend well in with a hand blender. Add the dry blend and blend completely with a hand blender.

Set it aside for 10–15 minutes while you preheat your broiler to 350° F. Rinse the material paper under warm water and shake it off before crushing it into your preparing tin, then add your blend to the tin and press it into the sides.

You can add nuts like almonds, sesame seeds, and pumpkin seeds to the highest point of the portion and pop it into the stove for 55 minutes.

Haul the bread out when completed and let it cool on a rack.

Nutrition:

Calories: 40 | Carbs: 4 g | Net Carbs: 2.5 g | Fibers: 5.5 g | Fats: 9 g | Proteins: 6 g

WHOLE WHEAT BREAD

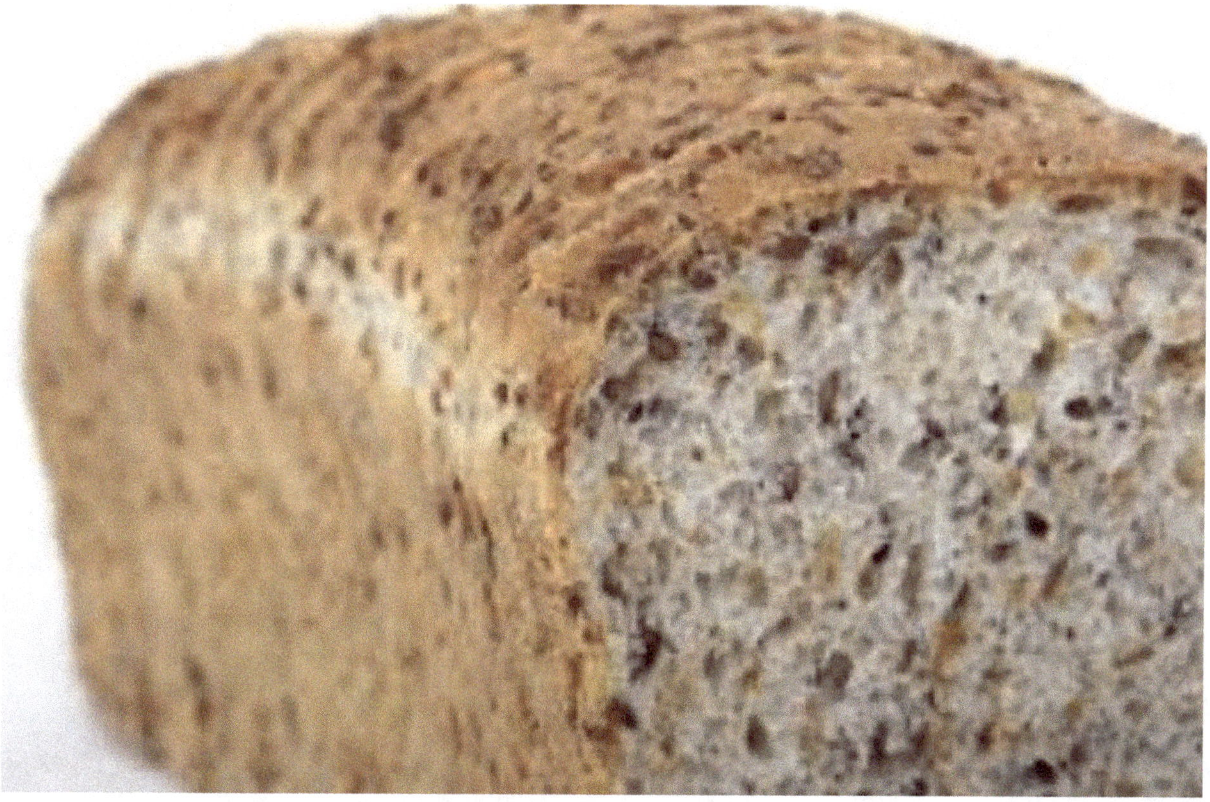

BREAD MACHINE EZEKIEL BREAD

Preparation Time: 10 minutes

Cooking Time: 3 hours

Servings: 12 slices

Ingredients:

¼ cup whole wheat flour

2 cups bread flour | ¼ cup spelled flour

1 tbsp. honey | 1 tbsp. millet

1 tbsp. olive oil | 1 tbsp. wheat germ

1 tbsp. dry kidney beans

1 tbsp. barley | 1 tbsp. dry lentils

1 tbsp. bread machine yeast

1 tbsp. dry black beans | ½ tsp salt

2 cups water at 90°F (320°C)

Directions:

Soak all beans and grains in separate bowls overnight. Boil the black beans, dry kidney beans for about 1 hour, and then add lentils, millet, and barley. Next, boil for 15 minutes more.

Assemble boiled ingredients in a food processor and mix until mashed.

Spread water into the bread machine pan, add 2 tbsp. of olive oil and honey, and then add the flour, wheat germ. In one corner, add salt in another one yeast and START the Dough cycle.

When the bread machine beeps, add the mash to the dough and press the Whole Wheat cycle. Enjoy!

Nutrition:

Calories: 192 | Carbs: 31 g | Fats: 5 g | Proteins: 6 g

HONEY-OAT-WHEAT BREAD

Preparation Time: 10 minutes

Cooking Time: 3 hours and 45 minutes

Servings: 16 slices

Ingredients:

Active dry yeast | 2 tbsp. sugar

2 cup water at 1100°F (450°C)

2 cup all-purpose flour

¼ cup whole wheat flour

1 cup rolled oats | 1 tbsp. powdered milk

½ tsp salt | 2 tbsp. honey

2 tbsp. vegetable oil

1 tbsp. butter softened | Cooking spray

Directions:

Place the following into the pan of a bread machine: yeast, sugar, and water. Let the yeast dissolve and foam for approximately 10 minutes. In the meantime, in a bowl, combine the all-purpose flour, powdered milk, whole wheat flour, salt, and rolled oats.

Pour the butter, honey, and vegetable oil into the yeast mixture. Then add the flour mixture on top. Choose the Dough cycle and then push the START button. Let the bread machine fully finish the process, which spans approximately 1 ½ hour.

Place the dough into a 9x5-inch loaf pan that's coated with cooking spray. Leave the bread to rise in a warm place for 1 hour. Preheat the oven.

Bake for approximately 35 minutes in the warmed oven until the top turns golden brown. Enjoy!

Nutrition:

Calories: 281 | Carbs: 45 g | Fats: 9 g | Proteins: 6 g

BUTTER UP BREAD

Preparation Time: 10 minutes

Cooking Time: 3 hours

Servings: 12 slices

Ingredients:

1 cup bread flour

2 tbsp. margarine, melted

2 tbsp. buttermilk at 1100°F (450°C)

1 tbsp. sugar

1 tbsp. active dry yeast

2 eggs, at room temperature

½ tsp salt

Directions:

Prepare the bread machine pan by adding buttermilk, melted margarine, salt, sugar, flour, and yeast in the order specified by your manufacturer.

Select Basic/White Setting and press START.

Once baked, transfer onto wire racks to cool before slicing. Enjoy!

Nutrition:

Calories: 231 | Carbs: 36 g | Fats: 6 g | Proteins: 8 g

CHEESE BREAD

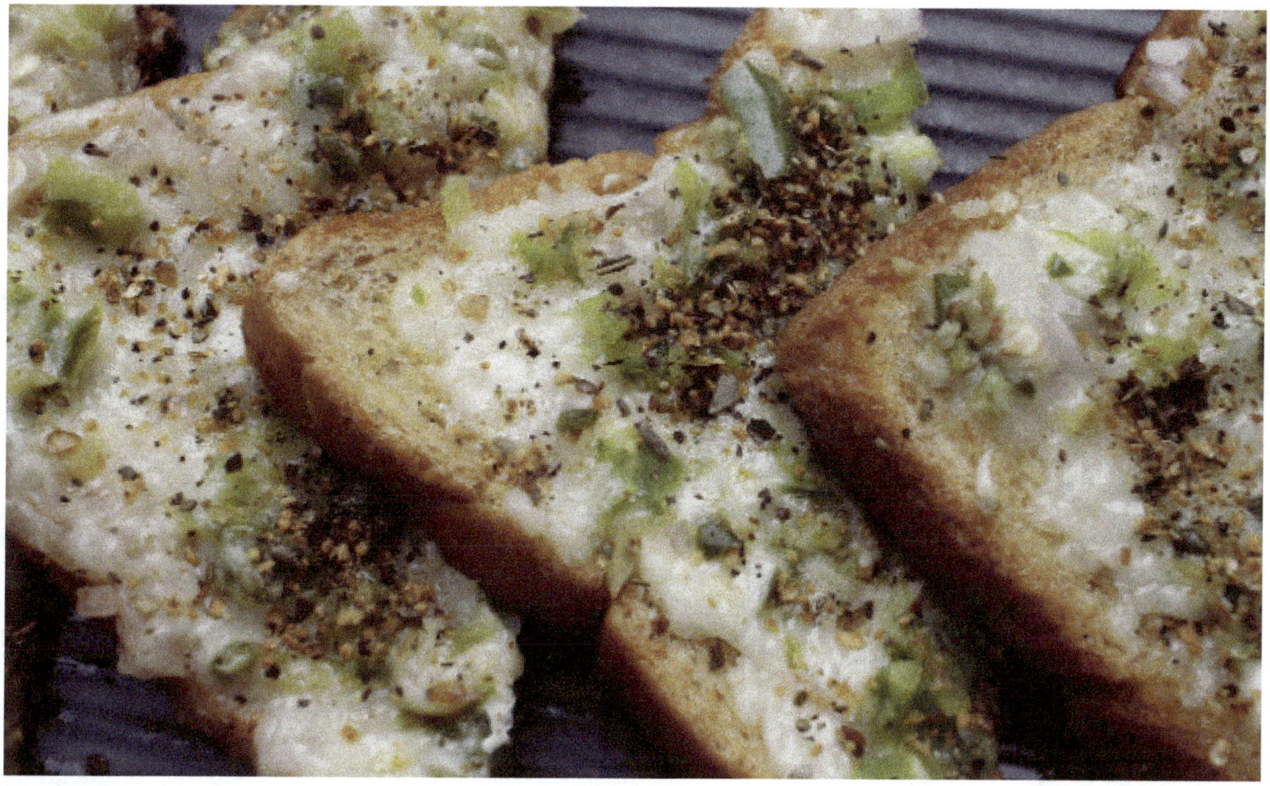

CHEESE PEPPERONI BREAD

Preparation Time: 5 minutes

Cooking Time: 2 hours

Servings: 10

Ingredients:

2/3 cup pepperoni, diced

1 ½ tsp. active dry yeast

3 ¼ cups bread flour

1 ½ tsp. dried oregano

1 ½ tsp. garlic salt

2 tbsp. sugar

1/3 cup. mozzarella cheese, shredded

1 cup+2 tbsp. warm water

Directions:

Add all ingredients except for pepperoni into the bread machine pan.

Select basic setting, then selects medium crust and press start.

Add pepperoni just before the final kneading cycle.

Once the loaf is done, remove the loaf pan from the machine.

Allow it to cool for 10 minutes. Slice and serve.

Nutrition:

Calories 176 | Carbs 34.5 g | Fats 1.5 g | Proteins 5.7 g

GLUTEN-FREE CHEESY BREAD

Preparation Time: 5 minutes

Cooking Time: 4 hours

Servings: 10

Ingredients:

3 eggs | 2 tbsp. olive oil

1 ½ cup water

2 ¼ tsp. active dry yeast

2 cups white rice flour

1 cup brown rice flour

¼ cup milk powder

2 tbsp sugar

1 tbsp. poppy seeds

3 ½ tsp. xanthan gum

1 ½ cup cheddar cheese, shredded

1 tsp. salt

Directions:

In a bowl, mix eggs, water, and oil and pour it into the bread machine pan.

In a large bowl, mix the other ingredients and pour over wet ingredient mixture into the bread pan. Select the whole wheat setting, then select light/medium crust and start.

Once the loaf is done, remove the loaf pan from the machine.

Allow it to cool for 10 minutes. Slice and serve.

Nutrition:

Calories 317 | Carbs 43.6 g | Fats 11 g | Proteins 10.6 g

GARLIC PARMESAN BREAD

Preparation Time: 5 minutes

Cooking Time: 3 hours and 45 minutes

Servings: 10

Ingredients:

¼ oz. active dry yeast

3 tbsp. sugar | 2 tsp. kosher salt

1 tsp. dried oregano

1 tsp. dried basil | ½ tsp. garlic powder

½ cup grated parmesan cheese

3 ½ cups all-purpose flour

1 tbsp. garlic, minced | ¼ cup butter, melted

1/3 cup olive oil | 1 and 1/3 cup water

Directions:

Add water, oil, butter, and garlic into the bread pan.

Add remaining ingredients except for yeast to the bread pan.

Make a small hole in the flour with your finger and add yeast to the spot.

Make sure yeast will not be mixed with any liquids.

Select the basic setting, then selects a light crust and start.

Once the loaf is done, remove the loaf pan from the machine.

Allow it to cool for 10 minutes. Slice and serve.

Nutrition:

Calories 335 | Carbs 37.7 g | Fats 15.4 g | Proteins 9.7 g

CHEESE JALAPENO BREAD

Preparation Time: 5 minutes

Cooking Time: 2 hours

Servings: 10

Ingredients:

¼ cup shredded Monterey jack cheese

2 tsp. Active dry yeast

1 ½ tbsp. butter | 1 ½ tbsp. sugar

3 tbsp. milk |3 cups flour

1 cup water

1 Jalapeno pepper, minced

1 ½ tsp. salt

Directions:

Begin by adding all fixings to the bread machine pan according to the bread machine manufacturer instructions.

Select basic bread setting, then select light/medium crust and start.

Once the loaf is done, remove the loaf pan from the machine.

Allow it to cool for 10 minutes. Slice and serve.

Nutrition:

Calories 174 | Carbs 31.1 g | Fats 3.1 g | Proteins 5.1 g

SPICE AND HERB BREAD

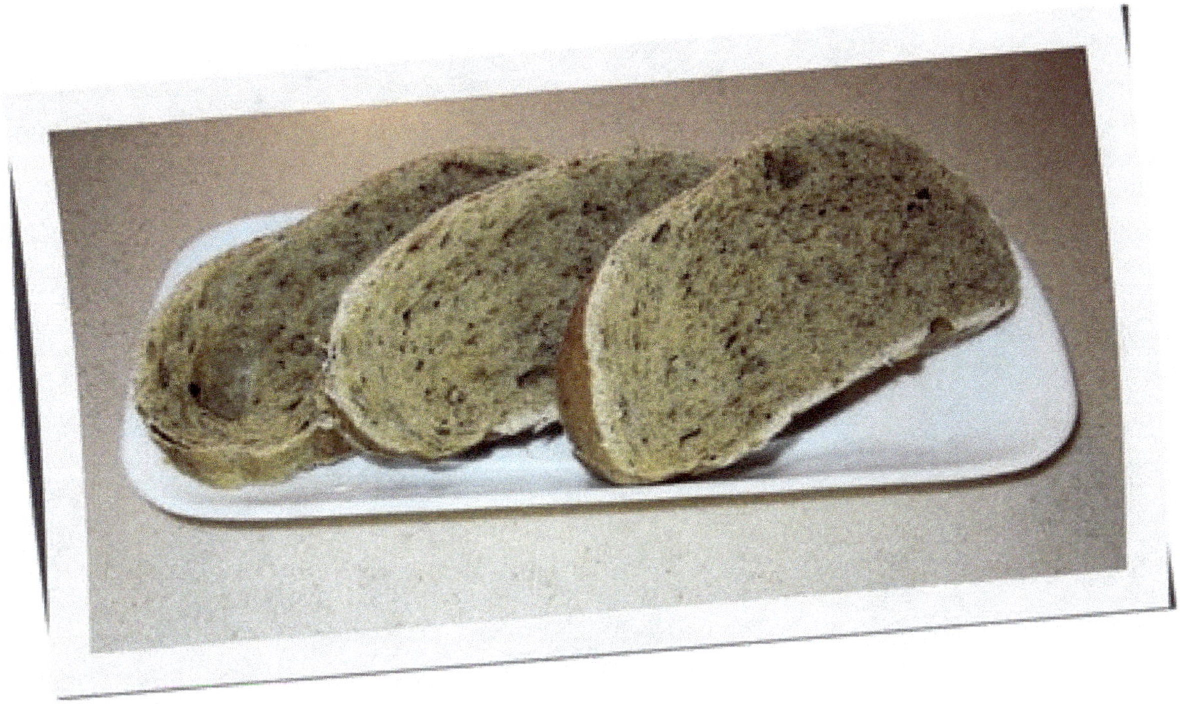

CAJUN BREAD

Preparation time: 10 minutes

Cooking time: 2 hours and 10 minutes

Servings: 14

Ingredients:

½ cup water

¼ cup chopped onion

¼ cup chopped green bell pepper

2 teaspoon finely chopped garlic

2 teaspoon soft butter

2 cups bread flour

1 tablespoon sugar

1 teaspoon cajun

½ teaspoon salt

1 teaspoon active dry yeast

Directions :

Add each ingredient to the bread machine in the order and at the temperature recommended by your bread machine manufacturer.

Close the lid, select the basic bread, medium crust setting on your bread machine and press start.

When the bread machine has finished baking, remove the bread and put it on a cooling rack.

Nutrition:

Carbs: 23 g | Fats: 4 g | Proteins: 5 g | Calories: 150

TURMERIC BREAD

Preparation time: 5 minutes

Cooking time: 3 hours

Servings: 14

Ingredients:

1 teaspoon dried yeast

4 cups strong white flour

1 teaspoon turmeric powder

2 teaspoons beetroot powder

2 tablespoons olive oil

1.5 teaspoon salt

1 teaspoon chili flakes

1 and 3/8 water

Directions:

Add each ingredient to the bread machine in the order and at the temperature recommended by your bread machine manufacturer.

Close the lid, select the basic bread, medium crust setting on your bread machine and press start.

When the bread machine has finished baking, remove the bread and put it on a cooling rack.

Nutrition:

Carbs: 24 g | Fats: 3 g | Proteins: 2 g | Calories: 129

ROSEMARY CRANBERRY PECAN BREAD

Preparation time: 30 minutes

Cooking time: 3 hours

Servings: 14

Ingredients:

1 and 1/3 cups water, plus

2 tablespoons water

2 tablespoons butter

2 teaspoons salt

4 cups bread flour

3/4 cup dried sweetened cranberries

3/4 cup toasted chopped pecans

2 tablespoons non-fat powdered milk

¼ cup sugar

2 teaspoons yeast

Directions:

Add each ingredient to the bread machine in the order and at the temperature recommended by your bread machine manufacturer.

Close the lid, select the basic bread, medium crust setting on your bread machine and press start.

When the bread machine has finished baking, remove the bread and put it on a cooling rack.

Nutrition:

Carbs: 18 g | Fats: 5 g | Proteins: 9 g | Calories: 120

SESAME FRENCH BREAD

Preparation time: 20 minutes

Cooking time: 3 hours and 15 minutes

Servings: 14

Ingredients:

7/8 cup water

1 tablespoon butter, softened

3 cups bread flour

2 teaspoons sugar

1 teaspoon salt

2 teaspoons yeast

2 tablespoons sesame seeds toasted

Directions:

Add each ingredient to the bread machine in the order and at the temperature recommended by your bread machine manufacturer.

Close the lid, select the French bread, medium crust setting on your bread machine and press start.

When the bread machine has finished baking, remove the bread and put it on a cooling rack.

Nutrition:

Carbs: 28 g | Fats: 3 g | Proteins: 6 g | Calories: 180

HERB BREAD

Preparation Time: 1 hour and 20 minutes

Cooking Time: 50 minutes (20+30 minutes)

Servings: 1 loaf

Ingredients:

3/4 to 7/8 cup milk

1 tablespoon sugar

1 teaspoon salt

2 tablespoons butter or margarine

1/3 cup chopped onion

2 cups bread flour

1/2 teaspoon dried dill

1/2 teaspoon dried basil

1/2 teaspoon dried rosemary

1 and 1/2 teaspoon active dry yeast

Directions:

Place all the Ingredients in the bread pan. Select medium crus then the rapid bake cycle.

Press starts. After 5-10 minutes, observe the dough as it kneads, if you hear straining sounds in your machine or if the dough appears stiff and dry, add 1 tablespoon liquid at a time until the dough becomes smooth, pliable, soft, and slightly tacky to the touch.

Remove the bread from the pan after baking.

Place on rack and allow to cool for 1 hour before slicing.

Nutrition:

Calories: 65 | Fats: 0 g | Carbohydrates: 13 g | Proteins: 2 g

VEGETABLE BREAD

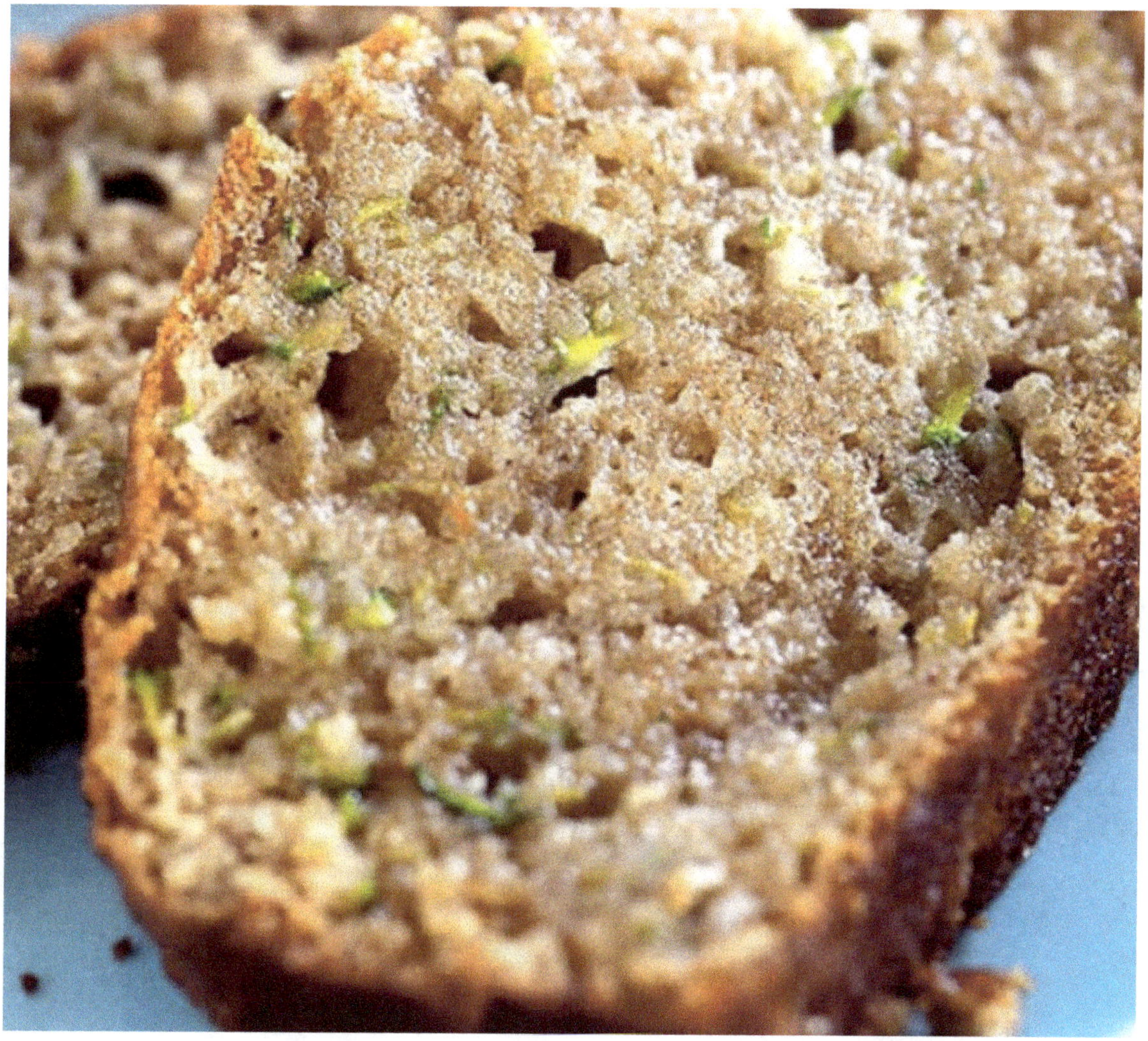

KETO SUNDRIED TOMATO QUICK BREAD

Preparation Time: 10 minutes

Cooking Time: 2 hours

Servings: 10

Ingredients:

2 ¼ cup almond flour

1 tbsp. baking powder

1 tsp. kosher salt

3 large eggs

1 ½ cup buttermilk

6 tbsp. canola oil

1 tbsp. dried basil

1 cup sundried tomato roughly chopped

Directions:

Place all the fixings in your bread machine bucket except for basil and sundried tomato.

Secure the lid cover. Select the QUICK BREAD setting on your bread machine then press START.

Wait for the ping or the fruit and nut signal to open the lid and add the basil and sundried tomato.

Place a cover and press START to continue.

When the cycle finishes, transfer the loaf to a wire rack and let it cool.

Slice and serve.

Nutrition:

Calories: 182 | Total Fats: 5.1 g | Cholesterol: 0 mg | Sodium: 318 mg | Protein: 2.7 g Total Carbohydrates: 31.3 g

FLAX SEED BREAD

Preparation time: 10 minutes

Cooking time: 20 minutes

Servings: 6

Ingredients:

2 cups flax seed, ground

1 tablespoon baking powder

1 and ½ cups protein isolate

A pinch of salt

6 egg whites, whisked

1 egg, whisked

¾ cup water

3 tablespoons coconut oil, melted

¼ cup stevia

Directions:

In a bowl, mix all dry ingredients and stir well.

In a separate bowl, mix the egg whites and the rest of the wet ingredients, stir well and combine the 2 mixtures.

Stir the bread and mix well. Pour into a loaf pan and bake at 350 degrees F for 20 minutes.

Cool the bread down, slice and serve.

Nutrition:

Calories 263 | Fats 17 g | Fibers 4 g | Carbs 2 g | Proteins 20 g

ALMOND BREAD WITH HAZELNUTS AND GARLIC

Preparation time: 25 minutes

Cooking time: 0 minutes

Servings: 8

Ingredients:

10 garlic cloves, chopped

1 cup of hazelnuts

3 cups of almond flour

2 teaspoons dry yeast

1 cup of garlic butter, melted

2 teaspoons sugar

10 tablespoons olive oil

2 cups of water

2 egg yolks | Sea salt to taste

Directions:

Preheat the oven to 300/320 degrees F and roast the hazelnuts in the oven for 10-15 minutes until lightly browned and crispy. Keep aside to cool wholly.

Blend the hazelnuts using a food processor. Melt the butter using a frying pan.

Chop the garlic cloves. Put the almond flour into the bowl and then add in the yeast, sugar, garlic, egg yolks, olive oil, and sea salt and mix until there is a smooth consistency.

Add in the hazelnuts. Spoon the mixture into the bread machine and add in the water and melted softened garlic butter, mix well.

Lubricate the surface of the dough with the water or the egg yolk.

Now close the lid and turn the bread machine on the basic/white bread program.

Allow to cool or place in refrigerator and then enjoy it.

Nutrition: Calories: 113 | Fats: 2 g | Carbohydrates 3.9 g | Proteins: 5 g

KETO ZUCCHINI BREAD

Preparation Time: 15 minutes

Cooking Time: 58 minutes

Servings: 12

Ingredients:

3 ounces almond flour

2 ounces coconut flour

1/2 teaspoon salt

1/2 teaspoon pepper

2 teaspoons heating powder

1 teaspoon thickener

5 enormous eggs

2/3 cup margarine dissolved

4 ounces cheddar ground

6 ounces zucchini ground and fluid crushed out

6 ounces bacon diced

Directions:

Preheat broiler to 175C/350F. In an enormous bowl include the almond flour, coconut flour, salt, pepper, preparing powder and thickener.

Blend well. Include the eggs and softened spread and blend well. Overlap through ¾ of the cheddar, alongside the zucchini and bacon.

Spoon into your lubed 9in clay portion dish (if utilizing a meat dish, line with material paper) and prepare for 35 minutes, expel from the stove and top with the rest of the cheddar.

Prepare for another 10-15 minutes, until the cheddar has caramelized and a stick confesses all. Leave to cool for 20 minutes. Cut into 12 cuts and appreciate warm.

Nutrition: Calories 270 | Fats 15 g | Fibers 3 g | Carbs 5 g | Proteins 9 g

KETO SPINACH BREAD

Preparation time: 10 minutes

Cooking time: 30 minutes

Servings: 10

Ingredients:

½ cup spinach, chopped

1 tablespoon olive oil

1 cup water

3 cups almond flour

A pinch of salt and black pepper

1 tablespoon stevia

1 teaspoon baking powder

1 teaspoon baking soda

½ cup cheddar, shredded

Directions:

In a bowl, mix the flour, with salt, pepper, stevia, baking powder, baking soda and the cheddar and stir well.

Add the remaining ingredients, stir the batter really well and pour it into a lined loaf pan.

Cook at 350 degrees F for 30 minutes, cool the bread down, slice and serve.

Nutrition:

Calories 142 | Fats 7 g | Fibers 3 g | Carbs 5 g | Proteins 6 g

HERBED GARLIC BREAD

Preparation time: 10 minutes

Cooking time: 45 minutes

Servings: 10

Ingredients:

½ cup coconut flour

8 tbsp. melted butter, cooled

1 tsp. baking powder

6 large eggs

¼ tsp. salt

1 tsp. garlic powder

1 tsp. rosemary, dried

½ tsp. onion powder

Directions:

Prepare bread machine loaf pan greasing it with cooking spray. In a bowl, add coconut flour, baking powder, onion, garlic, rosemary, and salt into a bowl.

Combine and mix well. Into another bowl, add eggs and beat until bubbly on top.

Add melted butter into the bowl with the eggs and beat until mixed.

Following the instructions on your machine's manual, mix the dry ingredients into the wet ingredients and pour in the bread machine loaf pan, taking care to follow how to mix in the baking powder.

Place the bread pan in the machine, and select the basic bread setting, together with the bread size and crust type, if available, then press start once you have closed the lid of the machine.

When the bread is ready, using oven mitts, remove the bread pan from the machine.

Let it cool before slicing. Cool, slice, and enjoy.

Nutrition: Calories 147 | Fats 12.5 g | Carbs 3.5 g | Proteins 4.6 g

SWEET BREAD

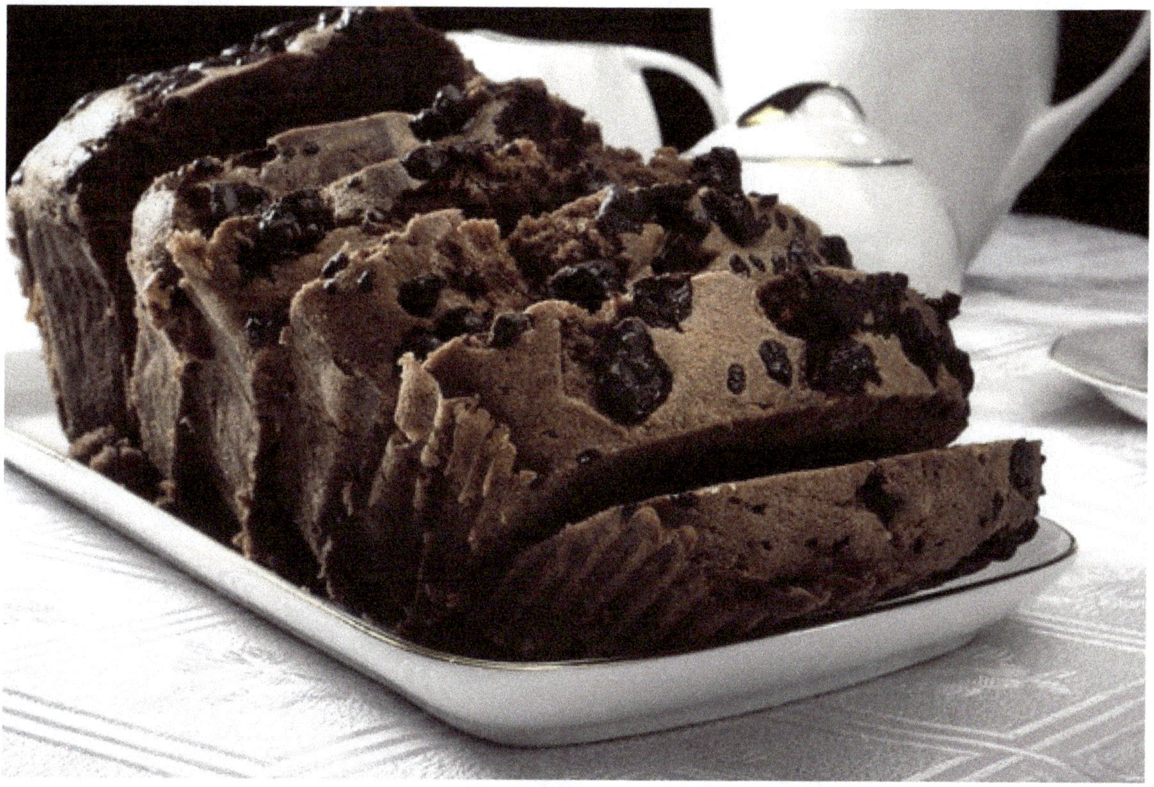

LEMON BREAD

Preparation time: 10 minutes

Cooking Time: 1 hour

Servings: 12 slices

Ingredients:

9.5 oz. (270 g) almond flour

½ tsp. keto baking powder

½ cup erythritol | 2 tbsp. poppy seeds

Zest of 2 lemons | 2 tbsp. lemon juice

3 tbsp. unsalted butter, melted

6 whole eggs

For Icing: ½ cup powdered erythritol

1 tbsp. lemon juice | 2 tbsp. water

Directions:

Prepare all of the ingredients for your bread and gather your measuring tools (a cup, a spoon, kitchen scales). Put all ingredients into the bread machine pan. Close the cover.

Set your bread machine program to CAKE. The time may vary depending on your device.

Press START. Help the machine to knead the dough, if necessary. After 40 minutes of baking, start checking for doneness using a toothpick.

The approximate baking time is 45 - 55 minutes.

Wait until the program is complete. When done, take the bucket out and let it cool for 5 - 10 minutes. Shake the loaf from the pan and let it cool for 30 minutes on a cooling rack.

Make the icing in a small bowl, mixing all the ingredients together. Drizzle it over the bread. Slice, serve, and enjoy the taste of fragrant lemon bread.

Nutrition:

Calories 193 | Net Carbs 12.9 g | Total Fats 17 g | Saturated Fats 3.4 g | Sodium 85 mg Cholesterol 89 g | Total Carbohydrates 15.6 g

HOLIDAY BREAD

Preparation time: 30 minutes

Cooking Time: 1 hour

Servings: 2 pounds / 12 slices

Ingredients:

2 ½ cups (250 g) almond flour

2 cups (140 g) whey isolate

1 cup (240 ml) lukewarm water

¼ cup (60 ml) almond milk

½ cup (100 g) powdered erythritol

½ cup (100 g) butter, melted

1 ½ tbsp. keto baking powder

2 tsp. xanthan gum | ½ tsp. sea salt

For Icing: ½ cup powdered erythritol

1 tbsp. lemon juice | 2 tbsp. water

Directions:

Prepare all of the ingredients for your bread and gather your measuring tools (a cup, a spoon, kitchen scales). Put all ingredients into the bread machine pan. Close the cover.

Set your bread machine program to CAKE. The time may vary depending on your device. Press START. Help the machine to knead the dough, if necessary. After 25 minutes of baking, start checking for doneness using a toothpick.

The approximate baking time is 30 - 35 minutes.

Wait until the program is complete. When done, take the bucket out and let it cool for 5 - 10 minutes. Shake the loaf from the pan and let it cool for 30 minutes on a cooling rack.

Make the icing in a small bowl, mixing all the ingredients together.

Drizzle it over the bread. Slice, serve, and enjoy the taste of fragrant sweet bread.

Nutrition:
Calories 130 | Net Carbs 5 g | Total Fats 11.8 g | Saturated Fats 6.1 g | Sodium 248 mg
Cholesterol 21 g | Total Carbohydrates 12 g

CINNAMON BREAD

Preparation time: 10 min

Cooking time: 4 hours

Servings: 2 pounds / 10 slices

Ingredients:

3 tablespoons sour cream

3 eggs, pasteurized

2 teaspoons vanilla extract, unsweetened

¼ cup / 60 grams melted butter, grass-fed, unsalted

2 cups / 200 grams almond flour

1/3 cup / 65 grams erythritol sweetener

2 tablespoons cinnamon

1 teaspoon baking soda

1 teaspoon baking powder

Directions:

Gather all the ingredients for the bread and plug in the bread machine having the capacity of 2 pounds of bread recipe.

Take a large bowl, place sour cream in it and then beat in eggs, vanilla, and butter until combined. Take a separate large bowl, place flour in it, and then stir in sweetener, cinnamon, baking powder, and soda until mixed.

Add egg mixture into the bread bucket, top with flour mixture, shut the lid, select the "basic/white" cycle setting and then press the up/down arrow button to adjust baking time according to your bread machine; it will take 3 to 4 hours.

Then press the crust button to select light crust if available, and press the "start/stop" button to switch on the bread machine.

When the bread machine beeps, open the lid, then take out the bread basket and lift out the bread. Let bread cool on a wire rack for 1 hour, then cut it into ten slices and serve.

Nutrition: Calories 169 | Fats 5 g | Proteins 4 g | Carbs 2 g | Fibers 2 g | Net Carbs 14,5 g

LEMON RASPBERRY LOAF

Preparation time: 10 minutes

Cooking time: 4 hours

Servings: 2 pounds / 12 slices

Ingredients:

2 eggs, pasteurized | 4 tablespoons sour cream

1 teaspoon vanilla extract, unsweetened

1 teaspoon lemon extract, unsweetened

4 tablespoons butter, grass-fed, unsalted, melted

1/4 cup / 50 grams erythritol sweetener

2 tablespoons lemon juice

½ cup / 100 grams raspberries preserves

2 cups / 200 grams almond flour

1 ½ teaspoons baking powder

Directions:

Gather all the ingredients for the bread and plug in the bread machine having the capacity of 2 pounds of bread recipe.

Take a large bowl, place flour in it, and then stir in baking soda until mixed. Take a separate large bowl, crack eggs in it, beat in sour cream, extracts, butter, sweetener, and lemon juice until blended and then stir in raspberry preserve until just combined.

Add egg mixture into the bread bucket, top with flour mixture, shut the lid, select the "basic/white" cycle setting and then press the up/down arrow button to adjust baking time according to your bread machine; it will take 3 to 4 hours.

Then press the crust button to select light crust if available, and press the "start/stop" button to switch on the bread machine.

When the bread machine beeps, open the lid, then take out the bread basket and lift out the bread. Let bread cool on a wire rack for 1 hour, then cut it into twelve slices and serve.

Nutrition: Calories 171 | Fats 14 g | Proteins 5 g | Carbs 5 g |Fibers 2.4 g | Net Carbs 3 g

WALNUT BREAD

Preparation time: 10 minutes

Cooking time: 4 hours

Servings: 1 ½ pounds / 10 slices

Ingredients:

4 eggs, pasteurized

2 tablespoons apple cider vinegar

4 tablespoons coconut oil

1/2 cup / 120 ml lukewarm water

1 cup / 200 grams walnuts chopped

½ cup / 65 grams coconut flour

1 tablespoon baking powder

2 tablespoons psyllium husk powder

1/2 teaspoon salt

Directions:

Gather all the ingredients for the bread and plug in the bread machine having the capacity of 2 pounds of bread recipe.

Take a large bowl, crack eggs in it, beat in vinegar, oil, and water until blended and stir in walnuts until just mixed. Take a separate large bowl, place flour in it, and then stir in baking powder, husk powder, and salt until mixed.

Add egg mixture into the bread bucket, top with flour mixture, shut the lid, select the "basic/white" cycle setting and then press the up/down arrow button to adjust baking time according to your bread machine; it will take 3 to 4 hours.

Then press the crust button to select light crust if available, and press the "start/stop" button to switch on the bread machine.

When the bread machine beeps, open the lid, then take out the bread basket and lift out the bread. Let bread cool on a wire rack for 1 hour, then cut it into ten slices and serve.

Nutrition: Calories 201 | Fats 8 g | Proteins 6 g | Carbs 7.5 g | Fibers 5 g | Net Carbs 3 g

SAVORY BREAD

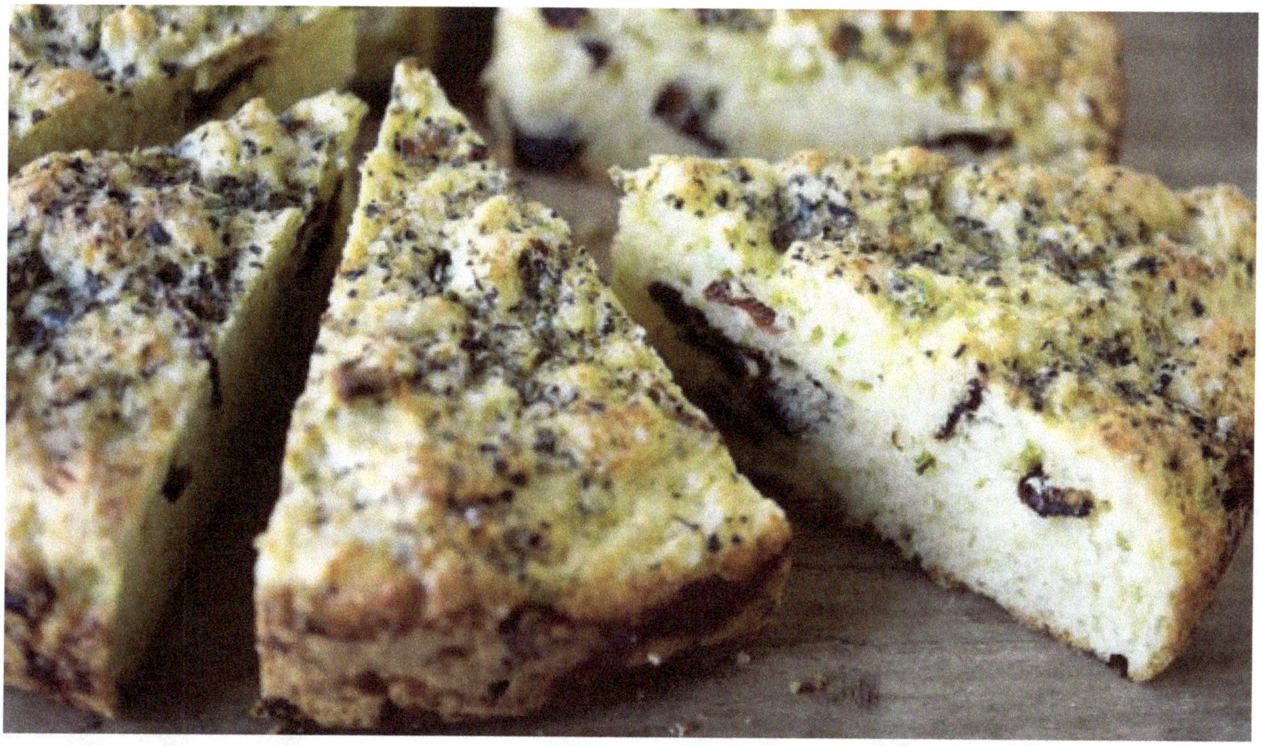

OLIVE BREAD

Preparation time: 10 minutes

Cooking time: 4 hours

Servings: 10 slices

Ingredients :

4 eggs

4 tbsp. avocado oil

1 tbsp. apple cider vinegar

½ cup coconut flour

1 tbsp. baking powder

2 tbsp. psyllium husk powder

1 ½ tbsp. dried rosemary

½ tsp. salt

1/3 cup black olives, chopped

½ cup boiling water

Directions :

Beat eggs, then blend in oil. Stir in vinegar and fold in the olives. In another bowl, place the flour, then stir in husk powder, baking powder, salt, and rosemary until mixed.

Add egg mixture into the bread bucket, top with flour mixture, and cover.

Select the Basic/White cycle or low-carb. Then press Start.

Remove the bread when done. Cool, slice, and serve.

Nutrition:

Calories: 85 | Fats: 6.5 g | Carbs: 3.4 g | Proteins: 2 g

JALAPEÑO CHEESE BREAD

Preparation time: 10 minutes

Cooking time: 4 hours

Servings: 8 slices

Ingredients :

2 tbsp. Greek yogurt, full-fat

4 eggs

1/3 cup coconut flour

½ tsp. sea salt

2 tbsp. whole psyllium husks

1 tsp. baking powder

¼ cup diced, pickled jalapeños

¼ cup shredded cheddar cheese, divided

Directions :

Beat yogurt and egg in a bowl. Place the flour in another bowl.

Add the remaining ingredients and mix well.

Add egg mixture into the bread bucket, top with flour mixture, and cover.

Select the Basic/White cycle or low-carb and press Start.

Remove the bread when done.

Cool, slice, and serve.

Nutrition:

Calories: 105 | Fats: 6.2 g | Carbs: 3.4 g | Proteins: 6.6 g

DILL AND CHEDDAR BREAD

Preparation time: 10 minutes

Cooking time: 4 hours

Servings: 10 slices

Ingredients :

4 eggs

¼ tsp. cream of tarter

5 tbsp. butter, unsalted

2 cups grated cheddar cheese

1 ½ cups almond flour

1 scoop of egg white protein

¼ tsp. salt

1 tsp. garlic powder

4 tsp. baking powder

¼ tbsp. dried dill weed

Directions :

Beat eggs, cream of tartar, butter, and cheese until just mixed.

Place flour in another bowl. Then stir in egg white protein, salt, garlic powder, baking powder, and dill and mix.

Add the egg mixture into the bread bucket, top with flour mixture.

Cover. Select the Basic/White cycle or low-carb and press Start.

Remove the bread when done. Cool, slice, and serve.

Nutrition:

Calories: 292 | Fats: 25.2 g | Carbs: 6.1 g | Proteins: 14.3 g

ITALIAN MOZZARELLA AND CREAM CHEESE BREAD

Preparation time: 10 minutes

Cooking time: 4 hours

Servings: 8 slices

Ingredients :

¾ cup shredded mozzarella cheese

¼ cup cream cheese, softened

1 egg

1/3 cup almond flour

¼ tsp. garlic powder

2 tsp. baking powder

½ tsp. Italian seasoning

½ cup shredded cheddar cheese

Directions :

Melt the mozzarella cheese and cream cheese in the microwave.

Beat the egg in another bowl.

Place flour in another bowl, add remaining ingredients, and mix.

Add blended egg into the bread bucket, top with melted cheese mixture, and then with flour mixture.

Cover. Select the Basic/White cycle or low-carb. Press Start.

Remove the bread when done.

Cool, slice, and serve.

Nutrition:

Calories: 171 | Fats: 14.5 g | Carbs: 1.5 g | Proteins: 3.3 g

SOURDOUGH DOUGH

Preparation time: 10 minutes

Cooking time: 4 hours

Servings: 15

Ingredients :

2 eggs | 6 egg whites

¾ cup coconut milk, unsweetened

¼ cup apple cider vinegar

½ cup of warm water (100F)

1 ½ cups almond flour

½ cup coconut flour

½ cup ground flaxseed

1 tsp. salt | 1 tsp. baking soda

1/3 cup psyllium powder

Directions :

In a bowl, add eggs, egg white, milk, vinegar, and water and whisk until combined.

In another bowl, place flour and stir in remaining ingredients until mixed.

Add the egg mixture into the bread bucket, top with flour mixture, and cover.

Select the Basic/White cycle or low-carb. Press Start.

Remove the bread when done.

Cool, slice, and serve.

Nutrition:

Calories: 115 | Fats: 8 g | Carbs: 4.7 g | Proteins: 5 g

CHEDDAR AND HERB BREAD

Preparation time: 10 minutes

Cooking time: 4 hours

Servings: 16 slices

Ingredients :

6 eggs | ½ tsp. salt

½ cup butter, unsalted, softened

2 cups almond flour

1 tsp. baking powder

½ tsp. xanthan gum

2 tbsp. garlic powder

1 tbsp. dried parsley

½ tbsp. dried oregano

1 ½ cups shredded cheddar cheese

Directions :

Beat eggs until frothy and then beat in the butter until combined.

Place flour in another bowl. Stir in remaining ingredients until mixed.

Add egg mixture into the bread bucket, top with flour mixture, and cover.

Select the Basic/White cycle or low-carb and press Start.

Remove the bread when done.

Cool, slice, and serve.

Nutrition:

Calories: 207 | Fats: 17.5 g | Carbs: 5 g | Proteins: 7.2 g

VEGETABLE LOAF

Preparation time: 10 minutes

Cooking time: 4 hours

Servings: 12 slices

Ingredients :

4 eggs | ¼ cup coconut oil

1 medium grated zucchini

1 cup grated pumpkin

1 small grated carrot

1/3 cup coconut flour

1 cup almond flour | 2 tsp. salt

2 tbsp. pumpkin seeds | 2 tbsp. flax seeds

2 tbsp. sunflower seeds | 2 tbsp. sesame seeds

2 tbsp. psyllium husks | 1 tbsp. smoked paprika

2 tsp. ground cumin | 2 tsp. baking powder

Directions :

Beat the eggs until frothy, beat in the oil, and then stir in zucchini, pumpkin, and carrot until just mixed. Place flour in another bowl.

Then stir in the remaining ingredients until mixed.

Add egg mixture into the bread bucket, top with flour mixture, and cover.

Select the Basic/White cycle or low-carb. Press Start.

Remove the bread when done. Cool, slice, and serve.

Nutrition:

Calories: 181 | Fats: 15 g | Carbs: 6.6 g | Proteins: 6.9 g

KETO ALMOND PUMPKIN QUICK BREAD

Preparation time: 10 minutes

Cooking time: 60 minutes

Servings: 16

Ingredients :

1/3 cup oil

3 large eggs

1 ½ cup pumpkin puree, canned

1 cup granulated sugar

1 ½ tsp. baking powder

½ tsp. baking soda

¼ tsp. salt

¾ tsp. ground cinnamon

¼ tsp. ground nutmeg

¼ tsp. ground ginger

3 cups almond flour

½ cup chopped pecans

Directions :

Grease the bread machine pan with cooking spray. Mix all the wet ingredients in a bowl.

Add all the dry ingredients except pecans until mixed. Pour the batter onto your bread machine pan and place it back inside the bread machine. Close and select Quick Bread.

Add the pecans after the beep. Remove the bread when done. Cool, slice, and serve.

Nutrition:

Calories: 54 | Fats: 13.3 g | Carbs: 6.3 g | Proteins: 9.6 g

KETO BASIL PARMESAN SLICES

Preparation time: 10 minutes

Cooking time: 3 hours and 25 minutes

Servings: 16 slices

Ingredients :

1 cup water

½ cup parmesan cheese, grated

3 tbsp. granulated sugar

1 tbsp. dried basil

1 ½ tbsp. olive oil

1 tsp. salt

3 cups almond flour

2 tsp. active dry yeast

Directions :

Place everything in the bread machine according to bread machine recommendation.

Select Basic and press Start.

Remove the bread when done.

Cool, slice, serve.

Nutrition:

Calories: 96 | Fats: 8 g | Carbs: 7 g | Proteins: 6 g

PROTEIN BREAD

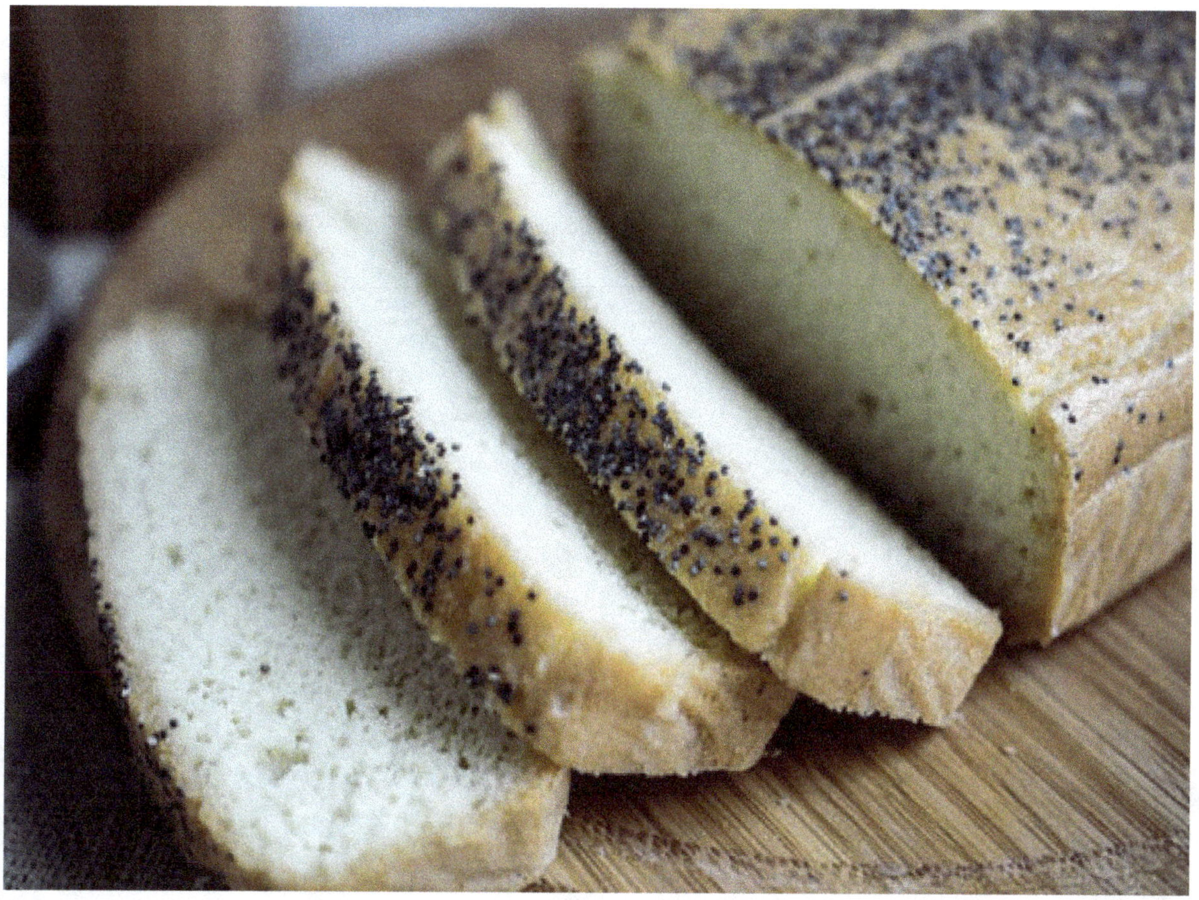

COCONUT FLOUR ALMOND BREAD

Preparation time: 10 minutes

Cooking time: 30 minutes

Servings: 4

Ingredients:

1 tbsp. butter, melted

1 tbsp. coconut oil, melted

6 eggs | 1 tsp. baking soda

2 tbsp. ground flaxseed

1 ½ tbsp. psyllium husk powder

5 tbsp. coconut flour

1 ½ cup almond flour

Directions:

Preheat the oven to 400F. Mix the eggs in a bowl for a few minutes.

Add in the butter and coconut oil and mix once more for 1 minute.

Add the almond flour, coconut flour, baking soda, psyllium husk, and ground flaxseed to the mixture. Let sit for 15 minutes.

Lightly grease the loaf pan with coconut oil. Pour the mixture in the pan.

Place in the oven and bake until a toothpick inserted in it comes out dry, about 25 minutes.

Nutrition:

Calories: 475 | Fats: 38 g | Carbs: 7 g | Proteins: 19 g

KETO CLOUD BREAD CHEESE

Preparation time: 5 minutes

Cooking time: 30 minutes

Servings: 12

Ingredients :

For cream cheese filling: 1 egg yolk

½ tsp. vanilla stevia drops for filling

8 oz. softened cream cheese

Base egg dough: ½ tsp. cream of tartar

1 tbsp. coconut flour

¼ cup unflavored whey protein

3 oz. softened cream cheese

¼ tsp. vanilla stevia drops for dough

4 eggs, separated

Directions:

Preheat the oven to 325F. Line two baking sheets with parchment paper.

In a bowl, stir the 8 ounces cream cheese, stevia, and egg yolk. Transfer to the pastry bag.

In another bowl, separate egg yolks from whites. Add 3 oz. cream cheese, yolks, stevia, whey protein, and coconut flour. Mix until smooth.

Whip cream of tartar with the egg whites until stiff peaks form. Fold in the yolk/cream cheese mixture into the beaten whites.

Spoon batter onto each baking sheet, 6 mounds on each.

Press each mound to flatten a bit. Add cream cheese filling in the middle of each batter.

Bake for 30 minutes at 325F.

Nutrition:

Calories: 120 | Fats: 10.7 g | Carbs: 1.1 g | Proteins: 5.4 g

MY KETO BREAD

Preparation time: 10 minutes

Cooking time: 50 to 60 minutes

Servings: 6

Ingredients:

3 egg whites

1 cup of boiling water

2 tbsp. sesame seeds

2 tsp. cider vinegar

1 tsp. sea salt

2 tsp. baking powder

5 tbsp. ground psyllium husk powder

1 ¼ cups almond flour

Directions:

Preheat the oven to 350F. Mix the dry ingredients in a bowl.

In another bowl, add the boiling water, vinegar, and egg whites.

Beat for 30 seconds with a hand mixer. Don't over mix.

Grease hands with oil to make 6 pieces then arrange on a greased baking sheet.

Bake 50 to 60 minutes in the lower rack of the oven.

Cooking time depends on the size of the bread.

The bread is ready when it makes a hollow sound when tapped.

Nutrition:

Calories: 170 | Fats: 13 g | Carbs: 2 g | Proteins: 7 g

KETO OAT CORNBREAD

Preparation time: 10 minutes

Cooking time: 20 minutes

Servings: 8

Ingredients:

¼ tsp. corn extract

4 eggs | ¼ cup water

1/3 cup melted bacon fat or coconut oil

4 oz. melted butter | ¼ tsp. salt

1 ½ tsp. baking powder

1/3 cup whey protein isolate, unflavored

½ cup oat fiber - ¼ cup coconut flour

Directions:

Preheat oven to 350F. Grease a 10-inch cast iron skillet and place in the oven to warm up.

Combine all the dry ingredients in a bowl.

Add the eggs, water, melted butter, and bacon fat.

Beat with a hand mixer, then mix in corn extract.

Transfer mixture into the heated skillet.

Bake at 350F for 18 to 20 minutes or until firm and top is lightly browned.

Nutrition:

Calories: 240 | Fats: 23 g | Carbs: 1 g | Proteins: 7 g

CHEESY KETO SESAME BREAD

Preparation time: 5 minutes

Cooking time: 30 minutes

Servings: 8

Ingredients:

1 tsp. sesame seeds

1 tsp. baking powder

1 tsp. salt

2 tbsp. ground psyllium husk powder

1 cup almond flour

4 tbsp. sesame or olive oil

7 ounces cream cheese

4 eggs | Sea salt

Directions:

Preheat the oven to 400F. Beat the eggs until fluffy.

Add cream cheese and oil until combined well.

Set the sesame seeds aside and add the remaining ingredients. Grease a baking tray.

Spread the dough in the greased baking tray. Allow it to stand for 5 minutes.

Baste dough with oil and top with a sprinkle of sesame seeds and a little sea salt.

Bake in the oven at 400F until the top is golden brown, about 30 minutes.

Nutrition:

Calories: 282 | Fats: 26 g | Carbs: 2 g | Proteins: 7 g

BREAD WITH BEEF AND PEANUTS

Preparation time: 3 hours

Cooking time: 20 minutes

Servings: 8

Ingredients :

15 oz. beef meat

5 oz. herbs de provence

2 big onions | 2 cloves chopped garlic

1 cup of milk | 20 oz. almond flour

10 oz. rye flour | 3 teaspoons dry yeast

1 egg | 3 tablespoons sunflower oil

1 tablespoon sugar | Sea salt

Ground black pepper | Red pepper

Directions :

Sprinkle the beef meat with the herbs de provence, salt, black, and red pepper and marinate in bear for overnight.

Cube the beef and fry in a skillet or a wok on medium heat until soft (for around 20 minutes). Chop the onions and garlic and then fry them until clear and caramelized.

Combine all the ingredients except for the beef and then mix well. Combine the beef pieces and the dough and mix in the bread machine.

Close the lid and turn the bread machine on the basic program.

Bake the bread until the medium crust and after the bread is ready take it out and leave for 1 hour covered with the towel and only then you can slice the bread.

Nutrition:

Carbohydrates 4 g | Fats 42 g | Proteins 27 g | Calories 369

BASIC SWEET YEAST BREAD

Preparation time: 3 hours

Cooking time: 20 minutes

Servings: 8

Ingredients :

1 egg | ¼ cup butter

1/3 cup sugar

1 cup milk

½ teaspoon salt

4 cups almond flour

1 tablespoon active dry yeast

After beeping: Fruits/ground nuts

Directions :

Add all of the ingredients to your bread machine, carefully following the instructions of the manufacturer (except fruits/ground nuts).

Set the program of your bread machine to basic/sweet and set crust type to light or medium. Press start. Once the machine beeps, add fruits/ground nuts.

Wait until the cycle completes. Once the loaf is ready, take the bucket out and let the loaf cool for 5 minutes.

Gently shake the bucket to remove loaf.

Transfer to a cooling rack, slice and serve. Enjoy!

Nutrition:

Carbohydrates 2.7 g | Fats 7.6 g | Protein 8.8 g | Calories 338

APRICOT PRUNE BREAD

Preparation time: 3 hours

Cooking time: 20 minutes

Servings: 8

Ingredients :

1 egg | 4/5 cup whole milk

¼ cup apricot juice | ¼ cup butter

1/5 cup sugar | 4 cups almond flour

1 tablespoon instant yeast

¼ teaspoon salt

5/8 cup prunes, chopped

5/8 cup dried apricots, chopped

Directions :

Add all of the ingredients to your bread machine, carefully following the instructions of the manufacturer (except apricots and prunes).

Set the program of your bread machine to basic/sweet and set crust type to light or medium. Press start. Once the machine beeps, add apricots and prunes.

Wait until the cycle completes. Once the loaf is ready, take the bucket out and let the loaf cool for 5 minutes.

Gently shake the bucket to remove loaf.

Transfer to a cooling rack, slice and serve. Enjoy!

Nutrition:

Carbohydrates 4 g | Fats 8.2 g | Proteins 9 g | Calories 364

CITRUS BREAD

Preparation time: 3 hours

Cooking time: 1 hour

Servings: 8

Ingredients :

1 egg | 3 tablespoons butter

1/3 cup sugar | 1 tablespoon vanilla sugar

½ cup orange juice | 2/3 cup milk

1 teaspoon salt | 4 cup almond flour

1 tablespoon instant yeast

¼ cup candied oranges

¼ cup candied lemon

2 teaspoons lemon zest

¼ cup almond, chopped

Directions :

Add all of the ingredients to your bread machine, carefully following the instructions of the manufacturer (except candied fruits, zest, and almond).

Set the program of your bread machine to basic/sweet and set crust type to light or medium. Press start. Once the machine beeps, add candied fruits, lemon zest, and chopped almonds. Wait until the cycle completes.

Once the loaf is ready, take the bucket out and let the loaf cool for 5 minutes.

Gently shake the bucket to remove loaf.

Transfer to a cooling rack, slice and serve. Enjoy!

Nutrition:

Carbohydrates 4 g | Fats 9.1 g | Proteins 9.8 g | Calories 404

CONCLUSION

Keto bread is not just another keto recipe. It's a balanced low carb bread that can be used as a meal replacement.Each of the issues is a suggestion that your body is in ketosis.

These are a few of the signs you will observe as you begin the transition:

You may experience keto flu or induction flu, which includes let down mental functions and energy. You may suffer from sleeping problems, bouts of nausea, augmented hunger, or other possible gastrointestinal worries. Several days into the keto plan should remedy these effects. If not, add ½ of a teaspoon of salt into a glass of water and drink it to help with the side effects. For the first week, you may need to do this daily. It could take up to 15 to 20 minutes before it helps. It will improve with time.

You may also notice an aroma similar to nail polish. Not surprising because this is acetone, a ketone product. It may also give you a unique body odor as your body adjusts to the diet changes. Maintain good oral health and use a breath refresher if needed.

Leg cramps may be an issue as you begin ketosis. The loss of magnesium (a mineral) can be a demon and create a bit of pain with the onset of the keto diet plan changes. With the loss of the minerals during urination, you could experience bouts of cramps in your legs.

Of course, the keto diet also has benefits that include:

Remain Satiated: Fat and protein are more filling and will stick to your ribs longer than products that are occupied with carbohydrates.

Dravet Syndrome: Dravet Syndrome is a severe form of epilepsy marked by prolonged, uncontrollable, and frequent seizures, which began in infancy. Unfortunately, available medications don't improve symptoms in approximately one-third of the Dravet Syndrome patients.

A clinical study used 13 children with Dravet Syndrome to stay on the ketogenic diet for more than one year to remain seizure-free. Over 50% of the group decreased in the frequency of the seizures. Six of the patients stopped the diet later, and one remains seizure-free.

Mental Focus: Your brain is approximately 60% fat by weight. By increasing your fatty food intake, you will have a better focus. It can maintain itself and work at total capacity.

Blood Pressure Levels Lowered: When you begin the ketogenic diet, your blood pressure may become lower, making you feel dizzy at first. Don't worry or feel overly concerned because that's a clear indication that the carbohydrates are working. However, if you are currently taking medications, it's a good idea to speak with your physician about the possibility of lowering some of your doses while on the ketogenic or intermittent fasting plan.

Polycystic Ovary Syndrome (PCOS): Young women of childbearing years can be affected by this disorder. It is further also associated with obesity, insulin resistance, and hyperinsulinemia. One study concluded a significant improvement in weight loss in fasting women over 24-weeks. The group limited carb intake to 20 grams daily for 24 weeks, which led to its success.

There are many more benefits, but you now have a good idea of how much better you can feel if you follow the keto techniques of dieting.

CPSIA information can be obtained
at www.ICGtesting.com
Printed in the USA
LVHW060739060422
715401LV00009B/404